A Colorful Journey into the World of Animals

Fun Facts for Curious Kids

Book 1: Mammals

Tena Nalker

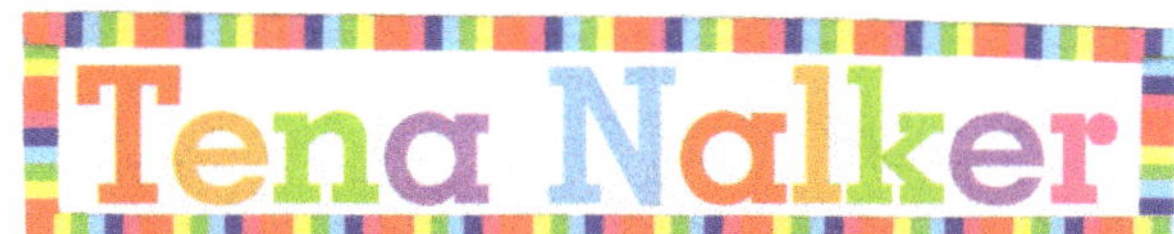

Archway Publishing books may be ordered through booksellers or by contacting:

Archway Publishing
1663 Liberty Drive
Bloomington, IN 47403
www.archwaypublishing.com
844-669-3957

ISBN: 978-1-6657-5623-5 (sc)
ISBN: 978-1-6657-5622-8 (hc)
ISBN: 978-1-6657-5621-1 (e)

Library of Congress Control Number: 2024902843

Print information available on the last page.

Archway Publishing rev. date: 02/23/2024

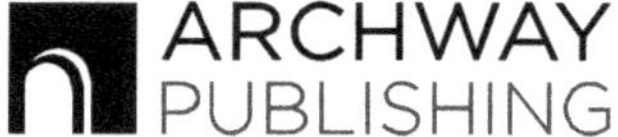

To my amazing husband, Daniel, who has always
encouraged me to follow my dreams!
And
to Bev, Laura, and Amarelis for offering
teacher pointers and encouragement!

I love you all!

Scientists

put all

Creatures

on

EARTH

into groups

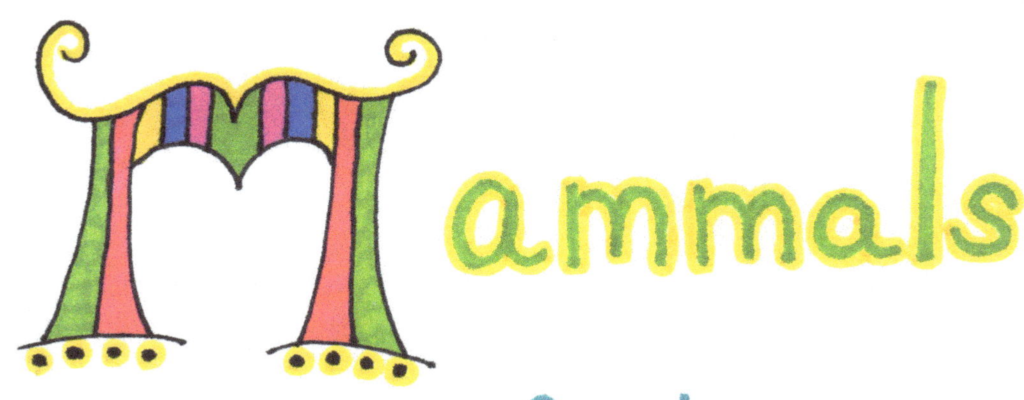

Mammals

are one of these groups. All mammals have seven common facts.

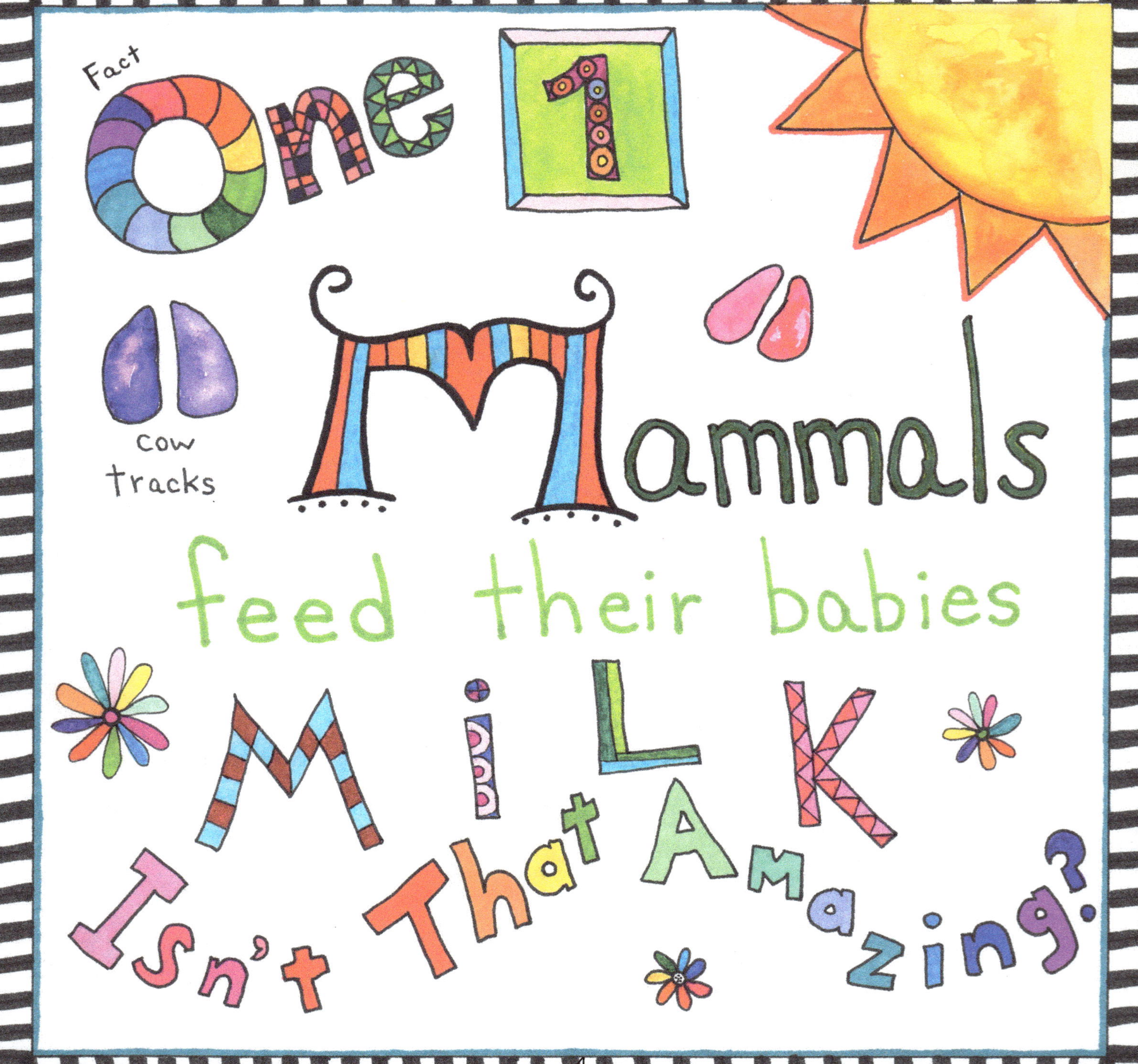
Fact
One 1
cow tracks
Mammals
feed their babies
MILK
Isn't That Amazing?

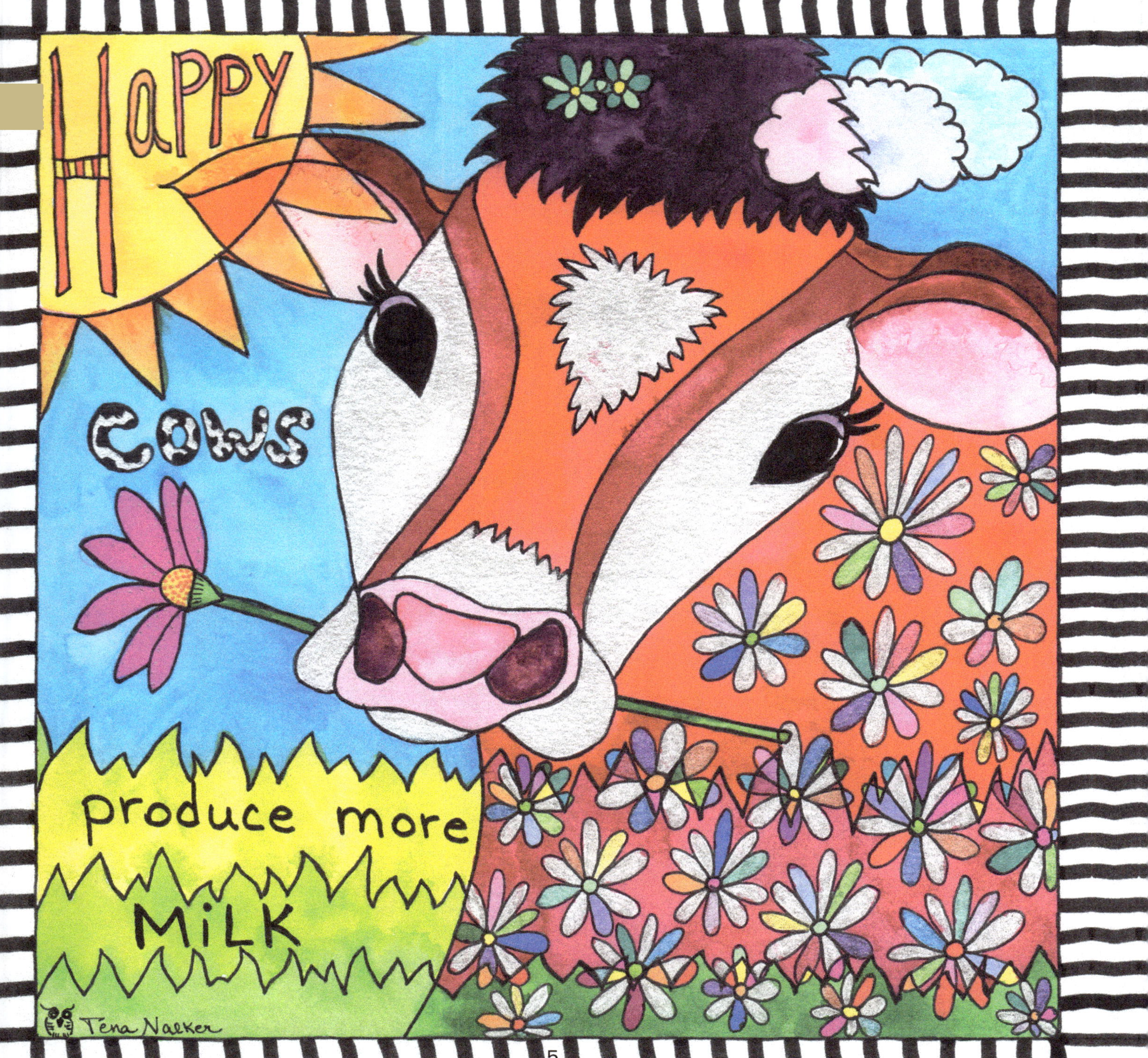

Happy
cows
produce more
MiLK
Tena Naeker
5

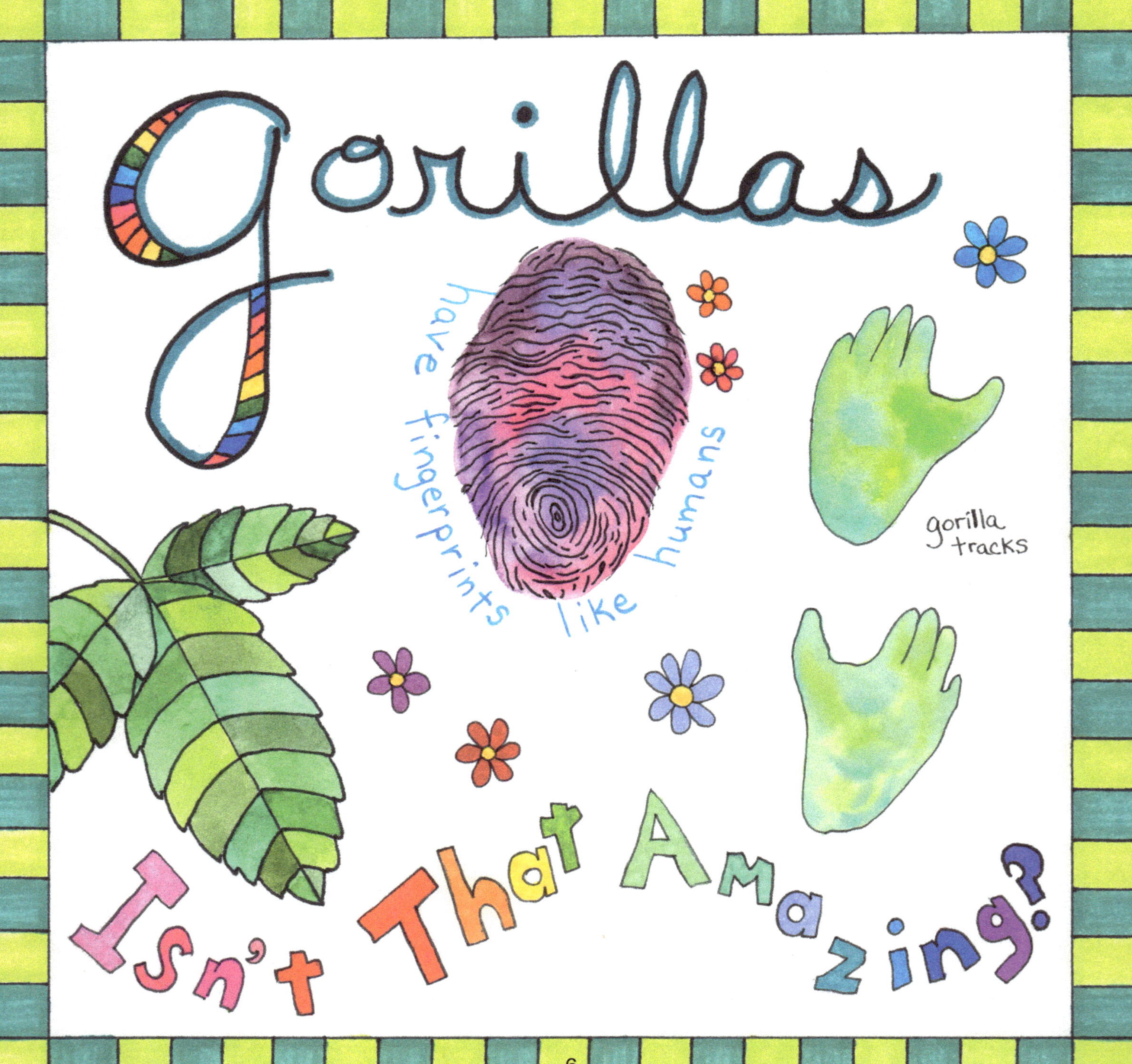
gorillas
have fingerprints like humans
gorilla tracks
Isn't That Amazing?

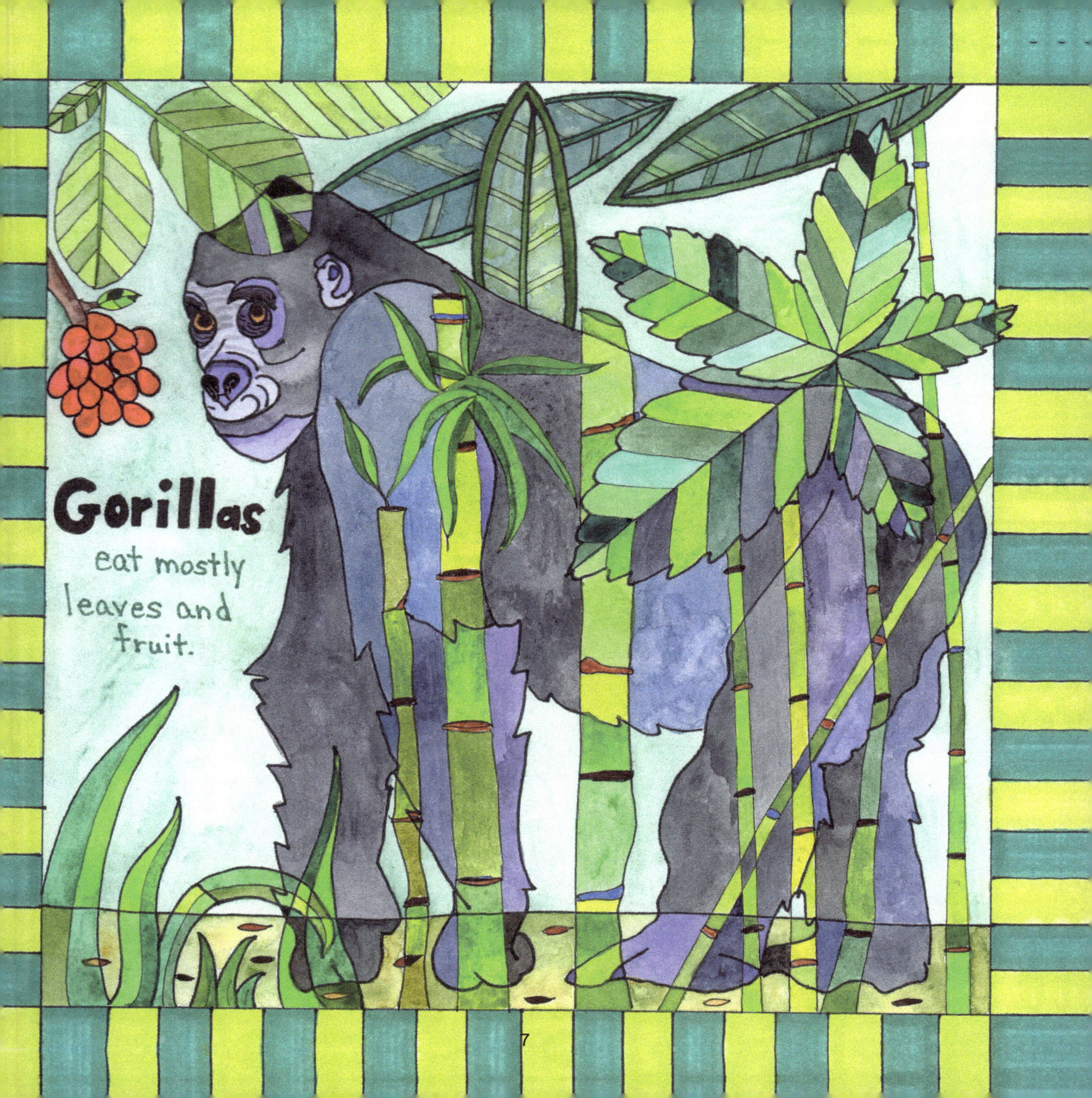

Gorillas
eat mostly leaves and fruit.

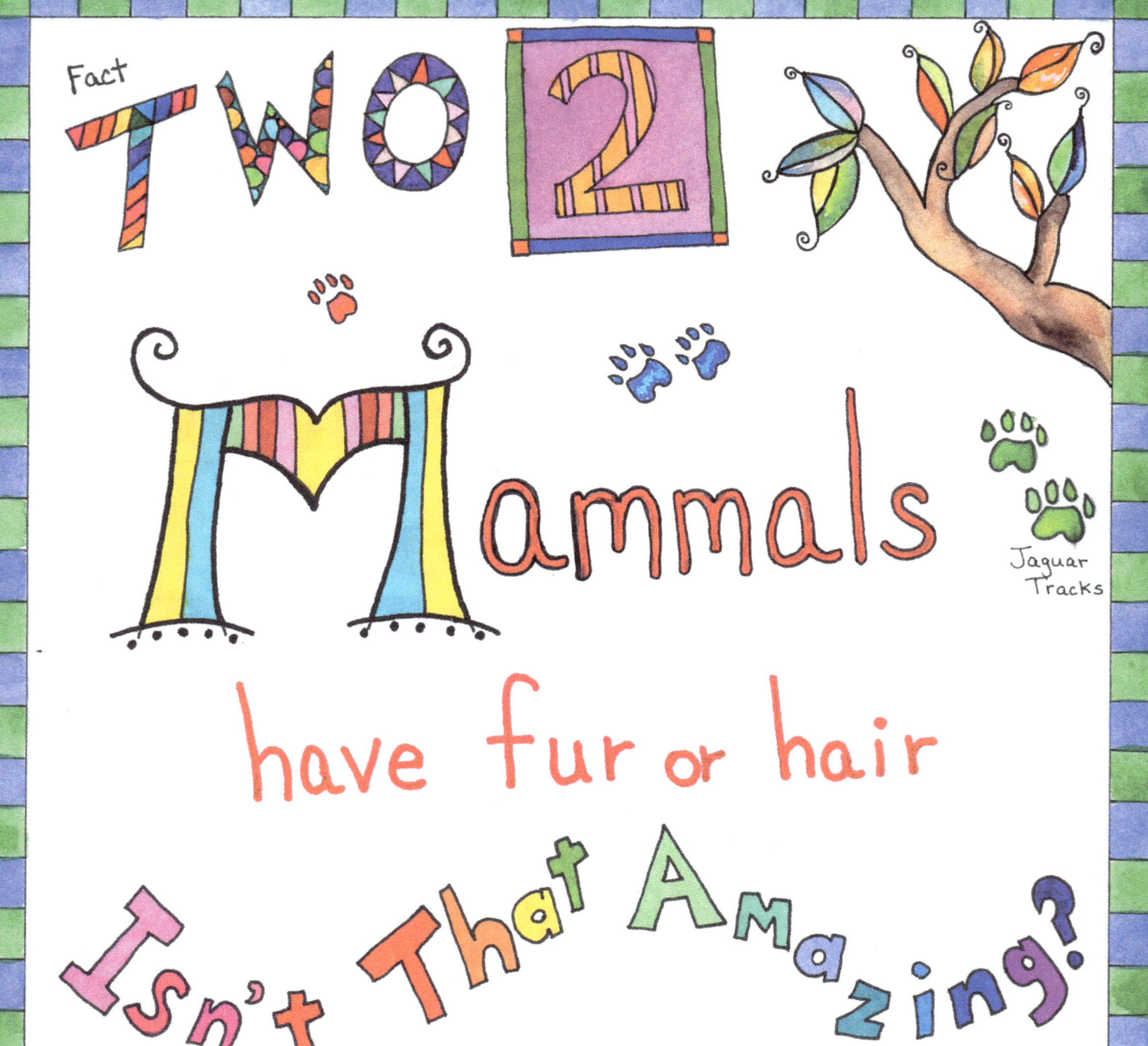
Fact
TWO 2
Mammals
have fur or hair
Isn't That Amazing?
Jaguar Tracks

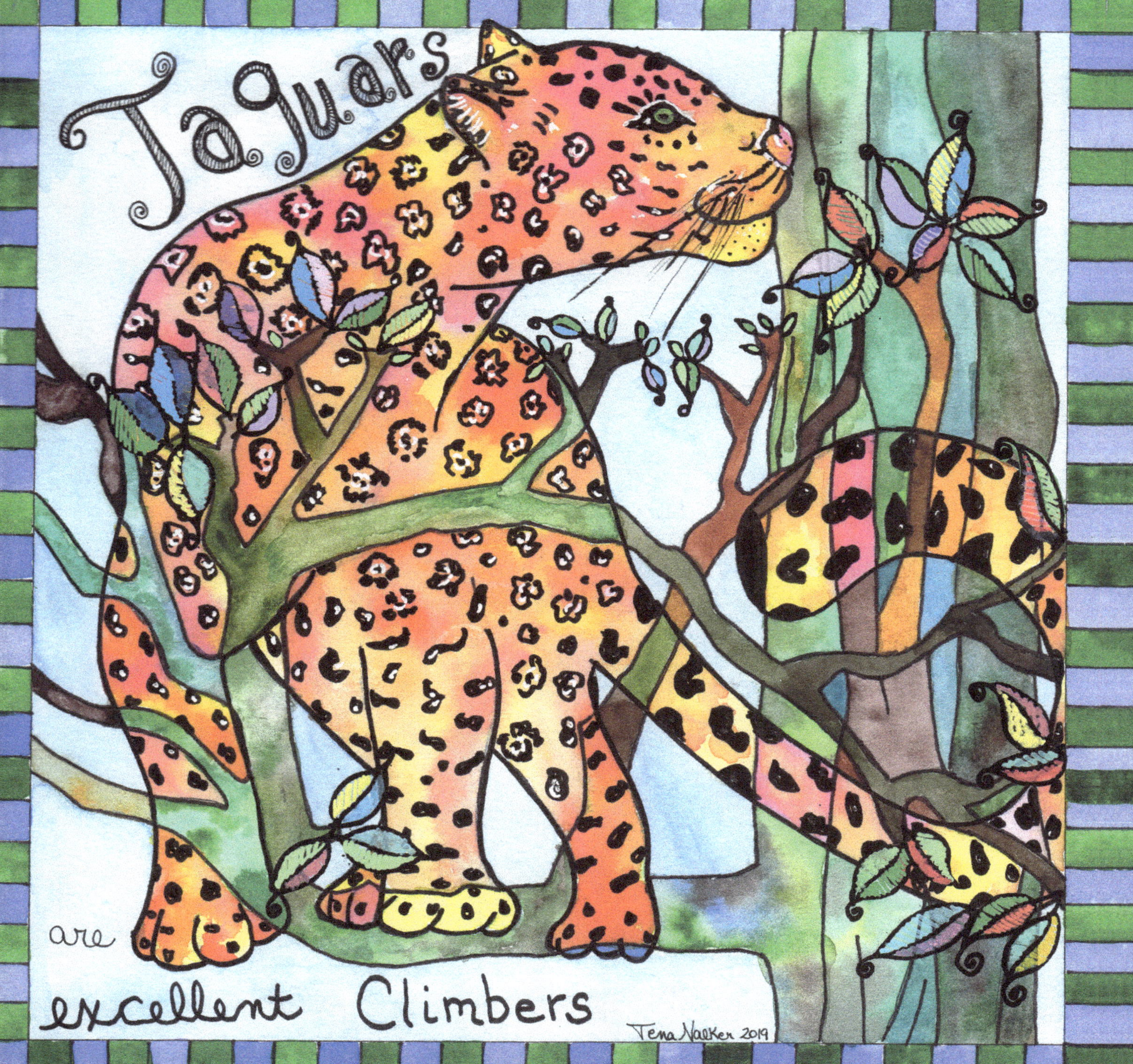

Jaguars
are
excellent Climbers
Tena Naeker 2019

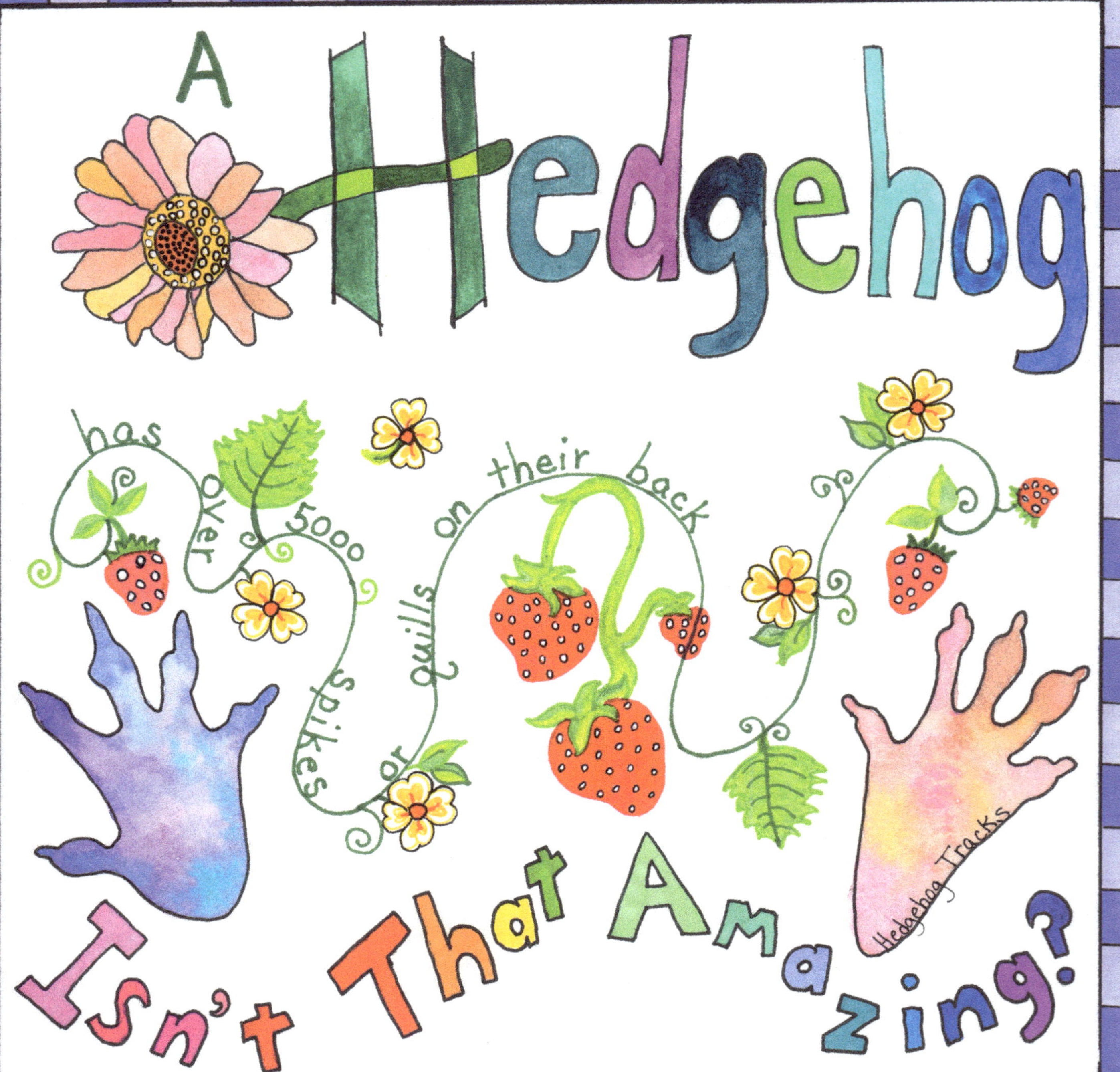
A Hedgehog
has over 5000 spikes or quills on their back
Isn't That Amazing?
Hedgehog Tracks

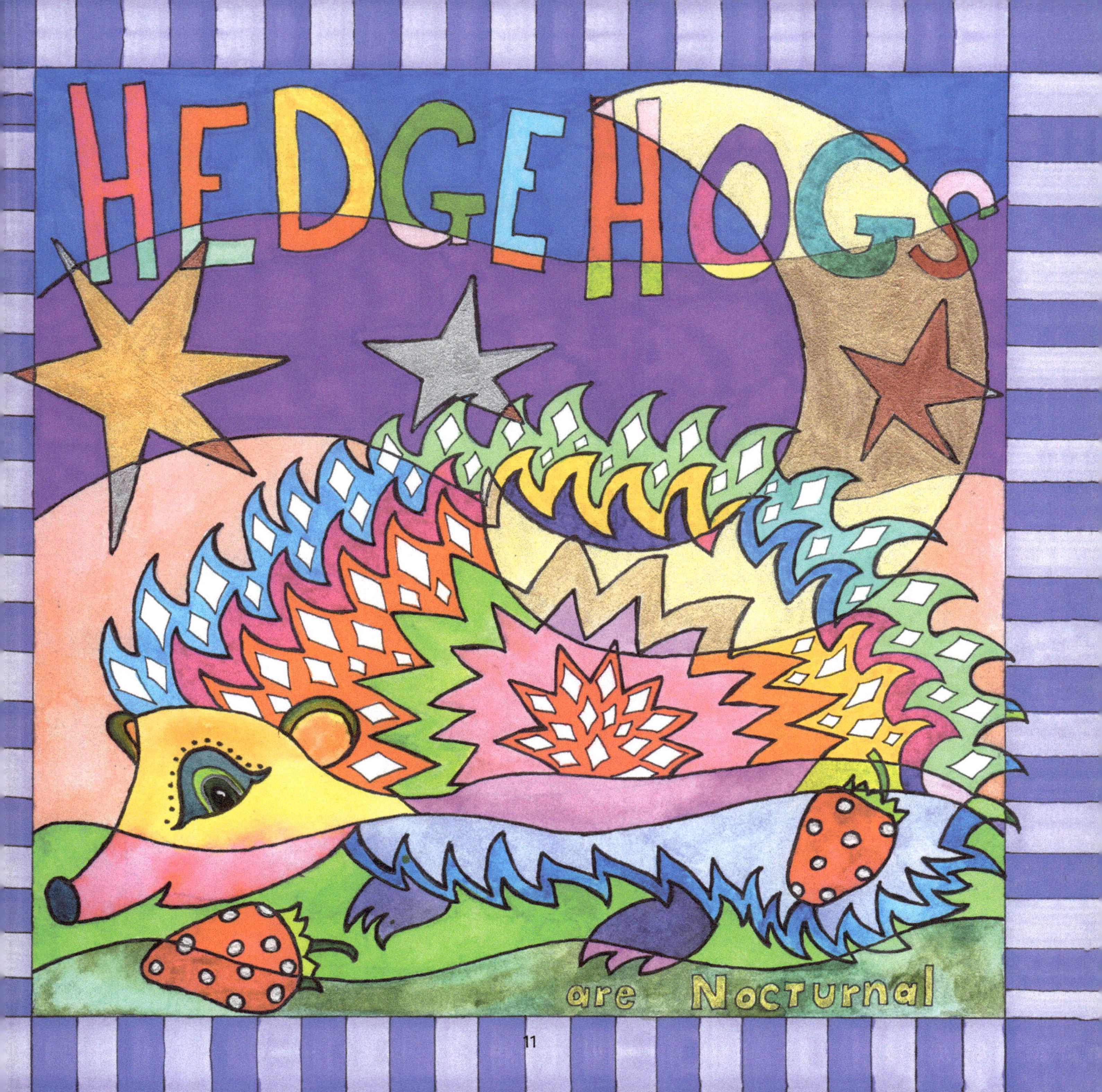

HEDGEHOGS
are Nocturnal

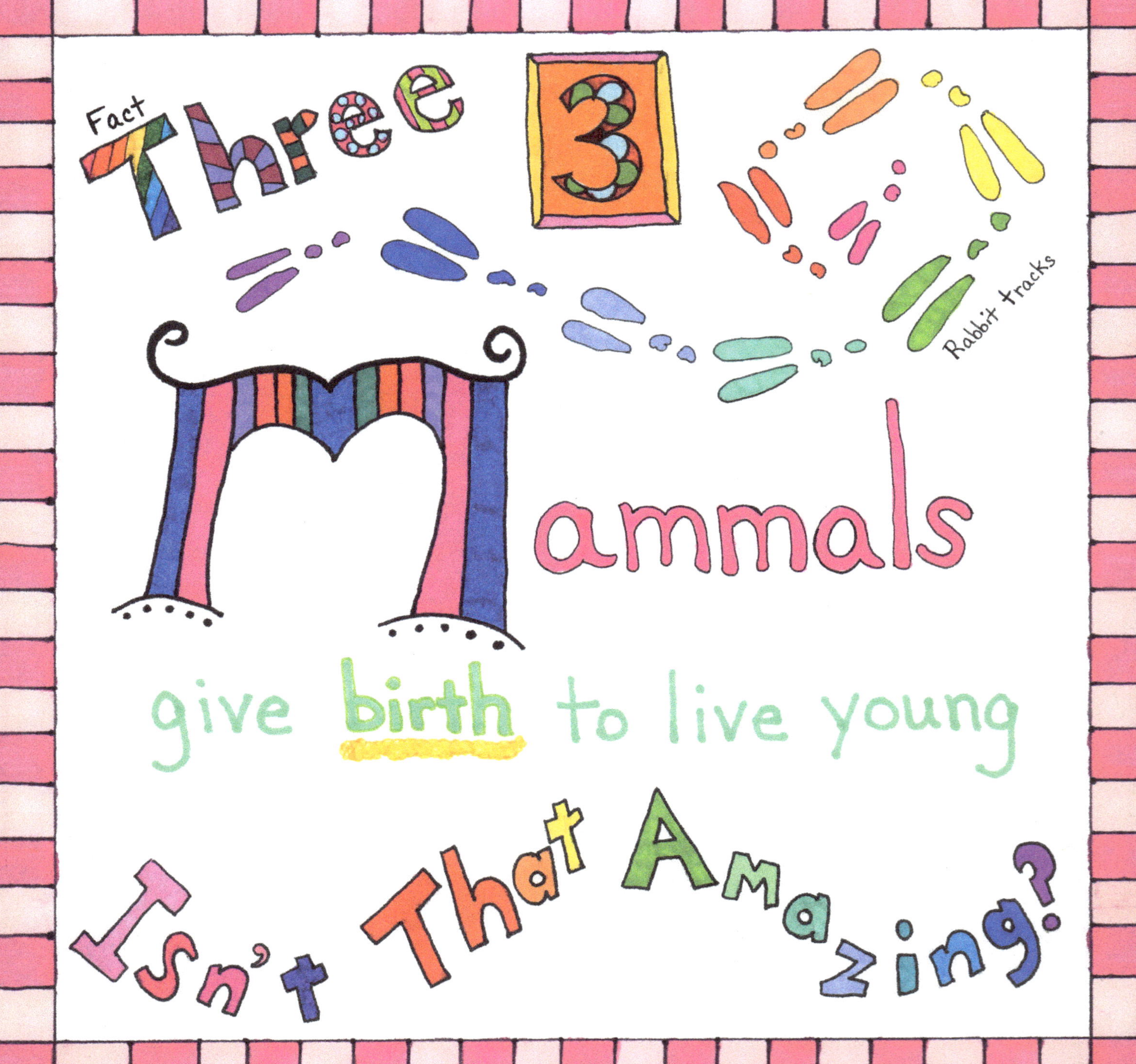

Fact Three 3
Rabbit tracks
Mammals
give birth to live young
Isn't That Amazing?

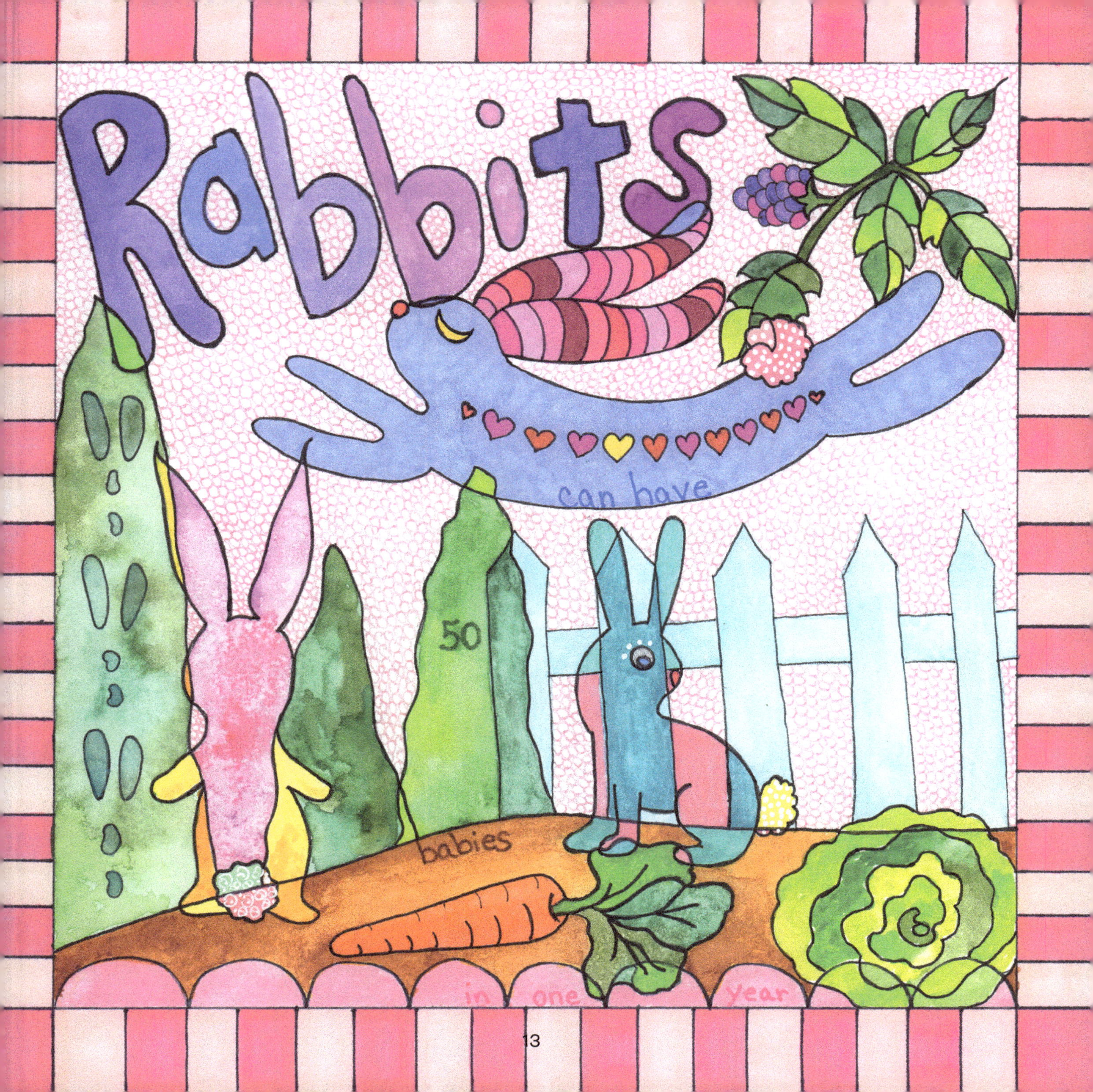

Rabbits
can have
50
babies
in one year
13

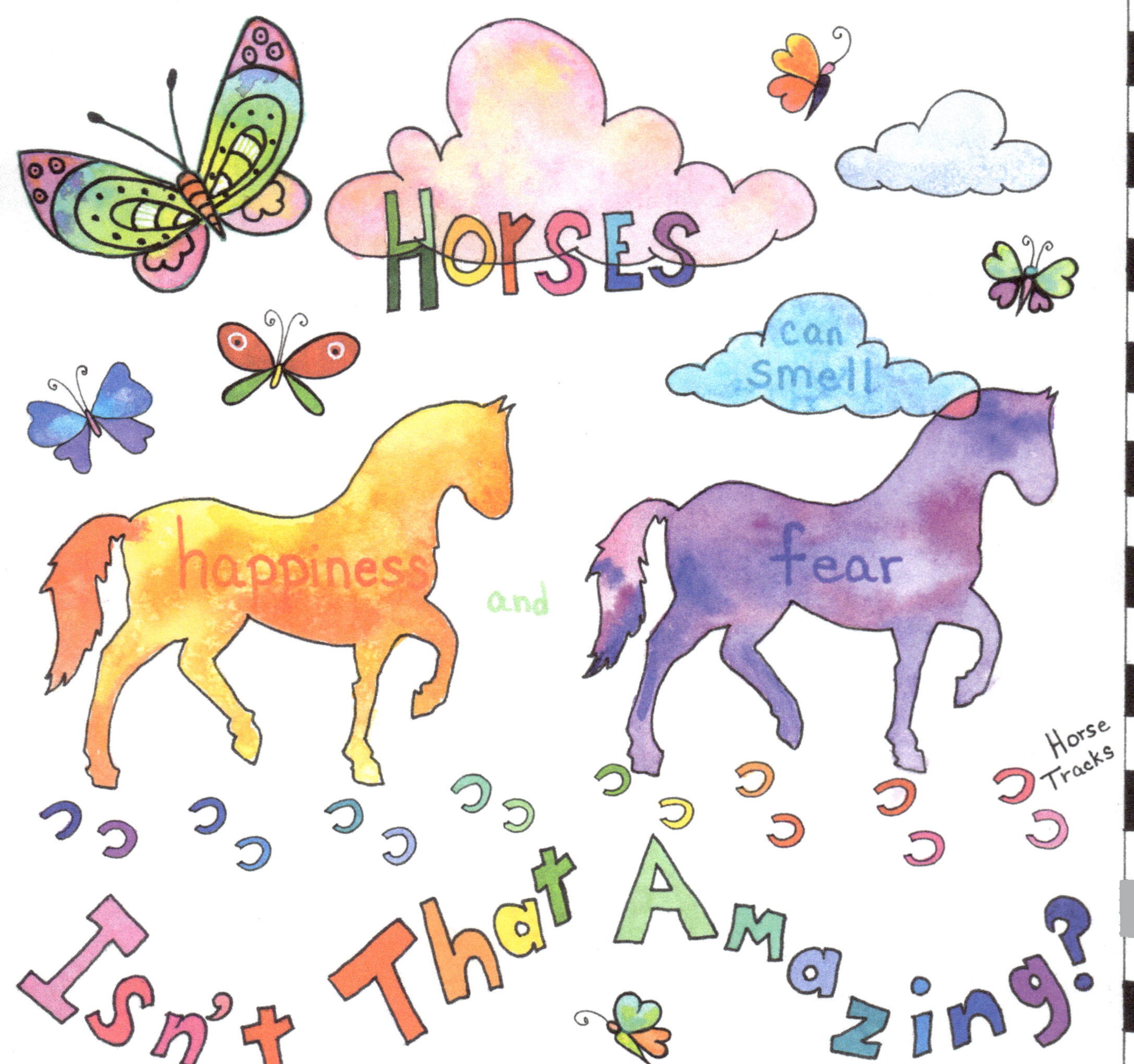
HORSES
can smell
happiness
and
fear
Horse Tracks
Isn't That Amazing?

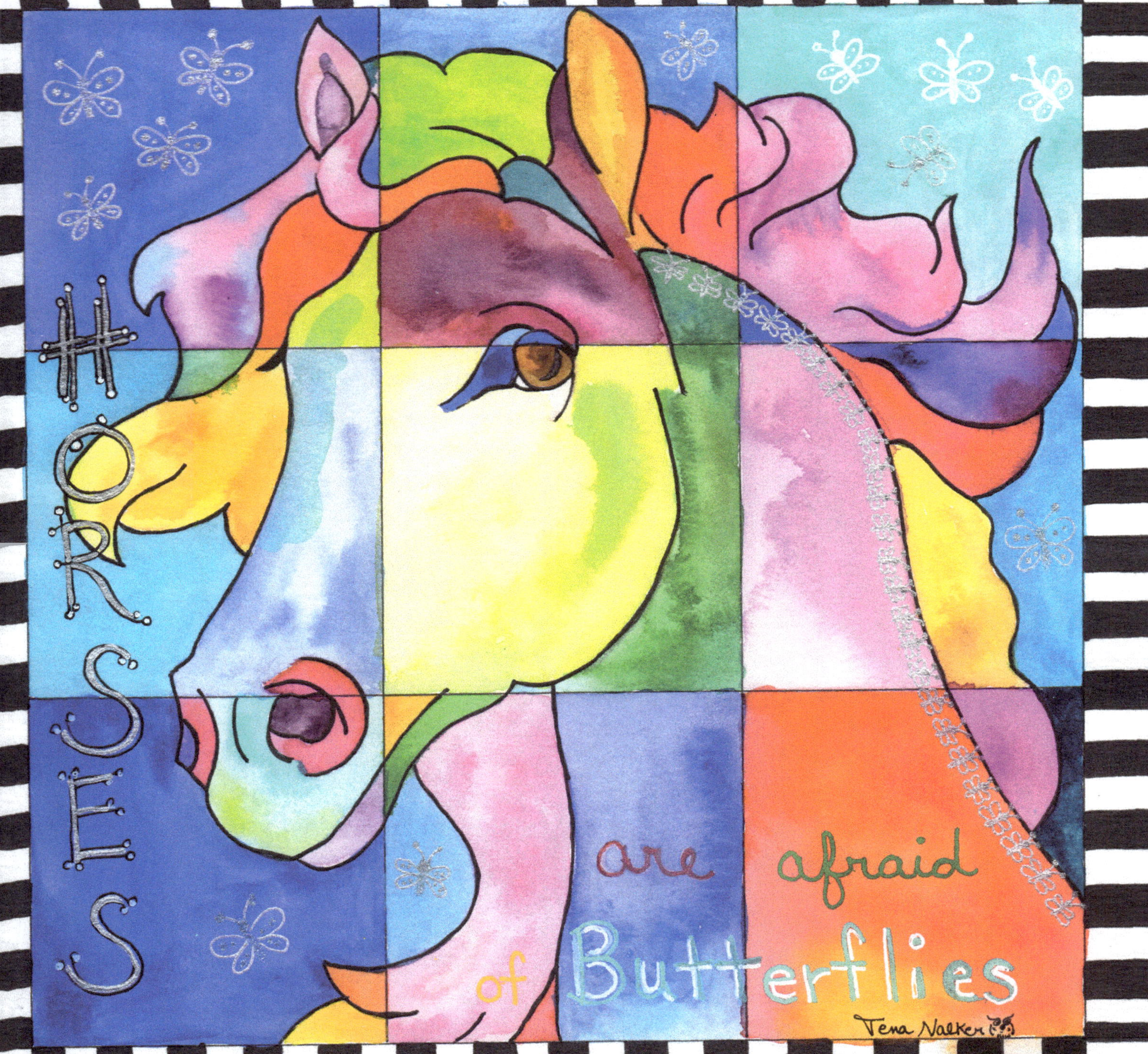
HORSES
are afraid
of Butterflies
Tena Nalker

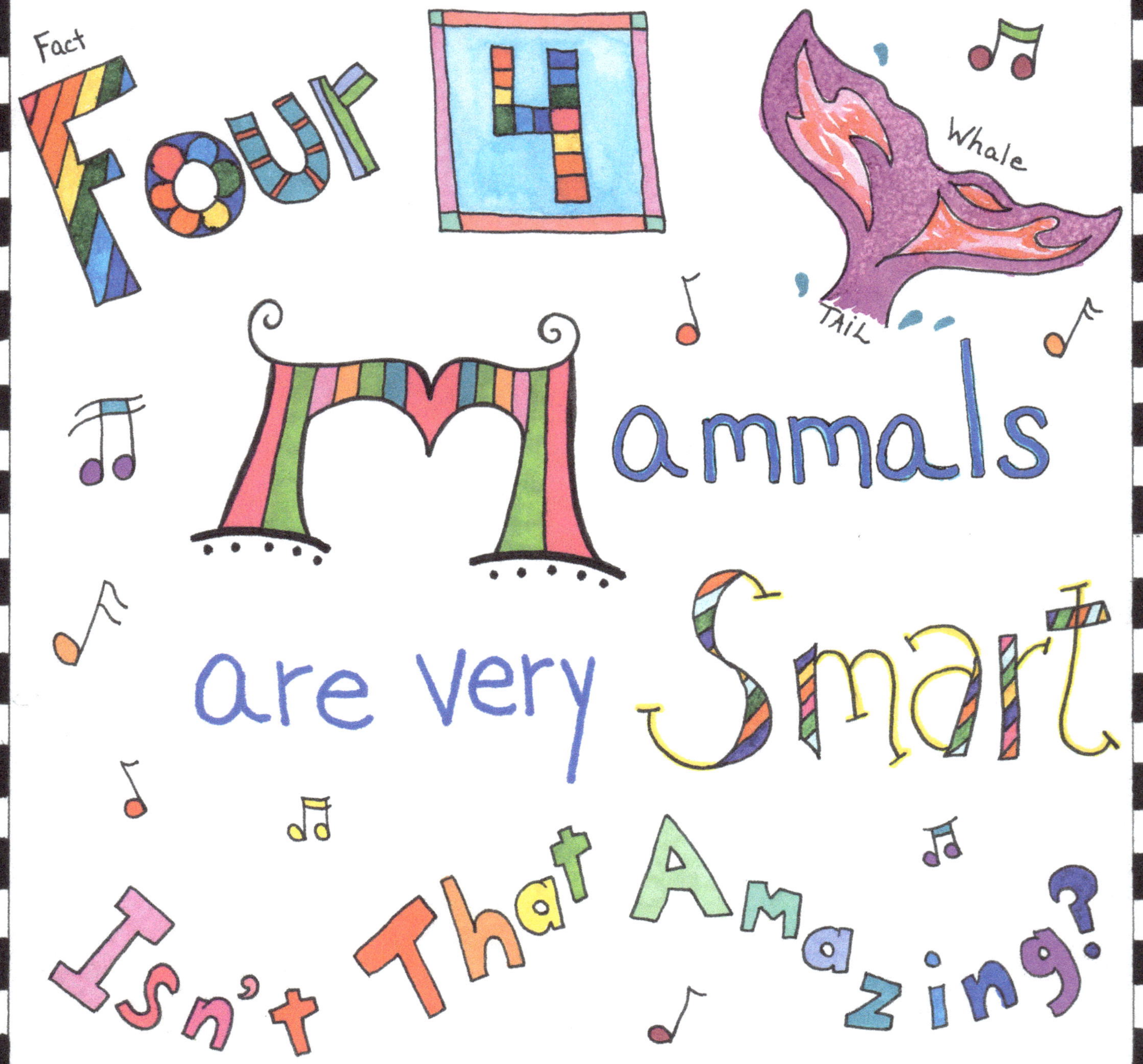

Fact
Four 4
Whale
TAiL
Mammals
are very Smart
Isn't That Amazing?

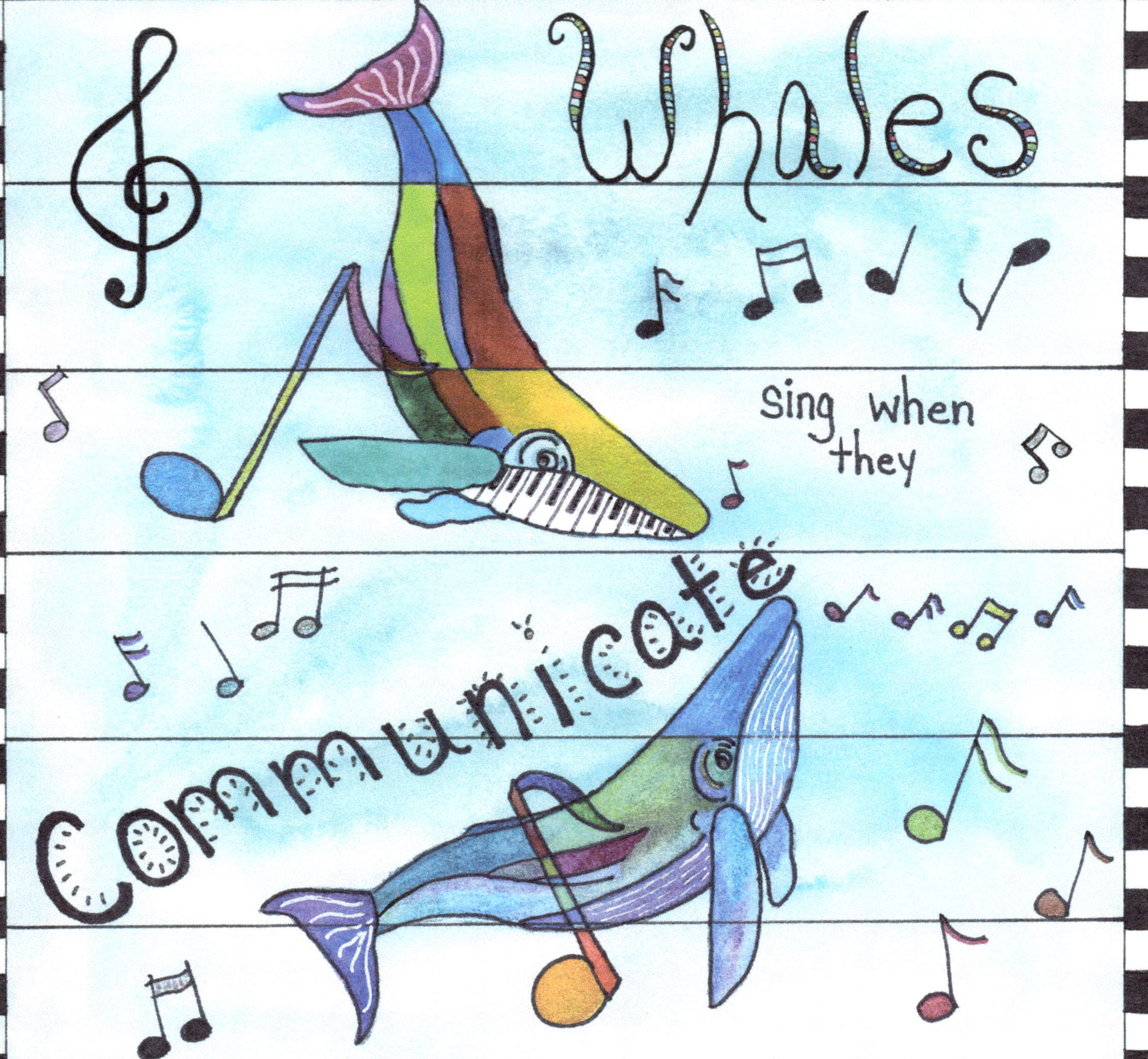

Whales
sing when they
Communicate
Jena Nasker 2019

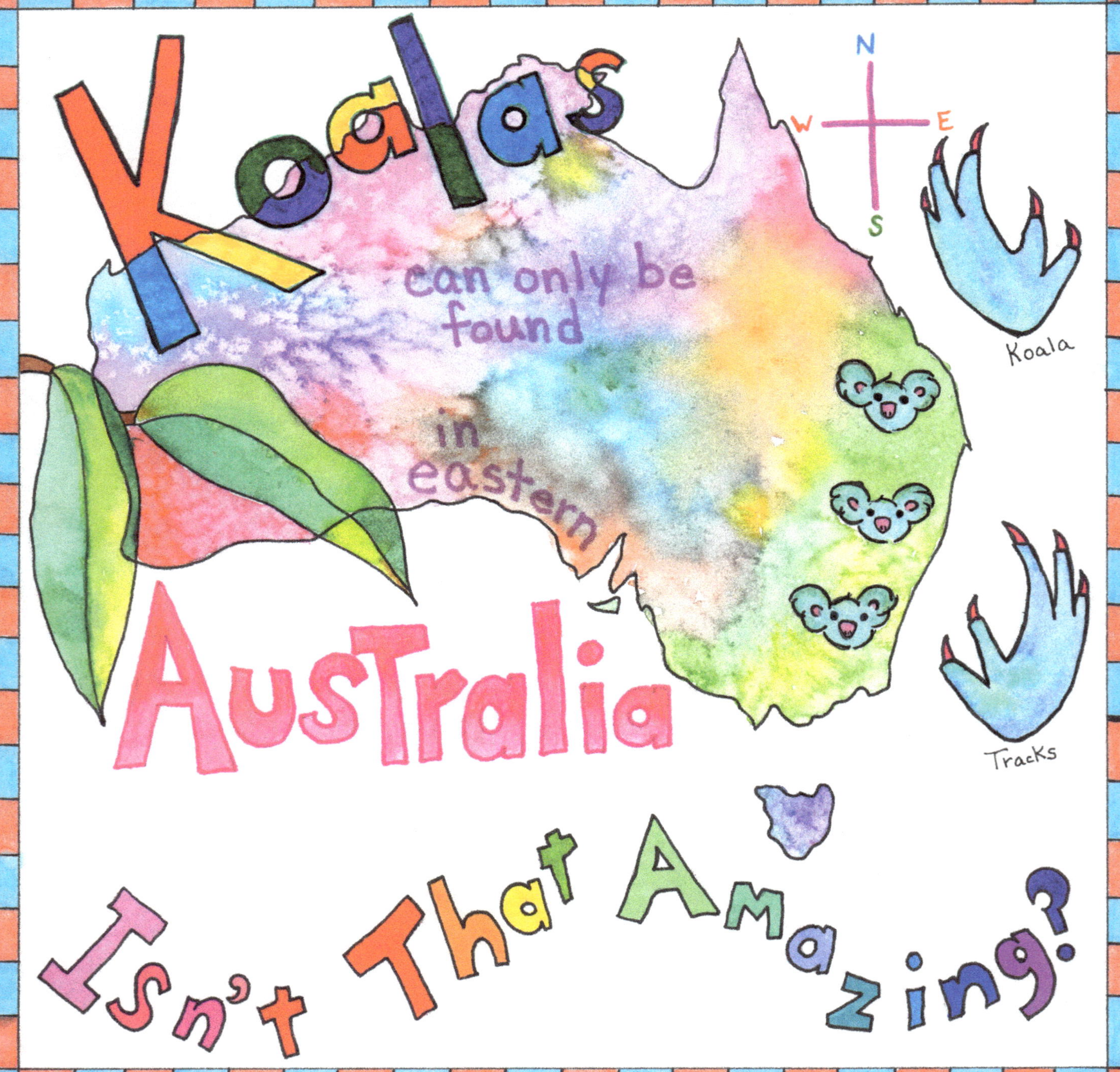

Koalas
can only be found
in eastern
Australia
Isn't That Amazing?
N
W
E
S
Koala
Tracks

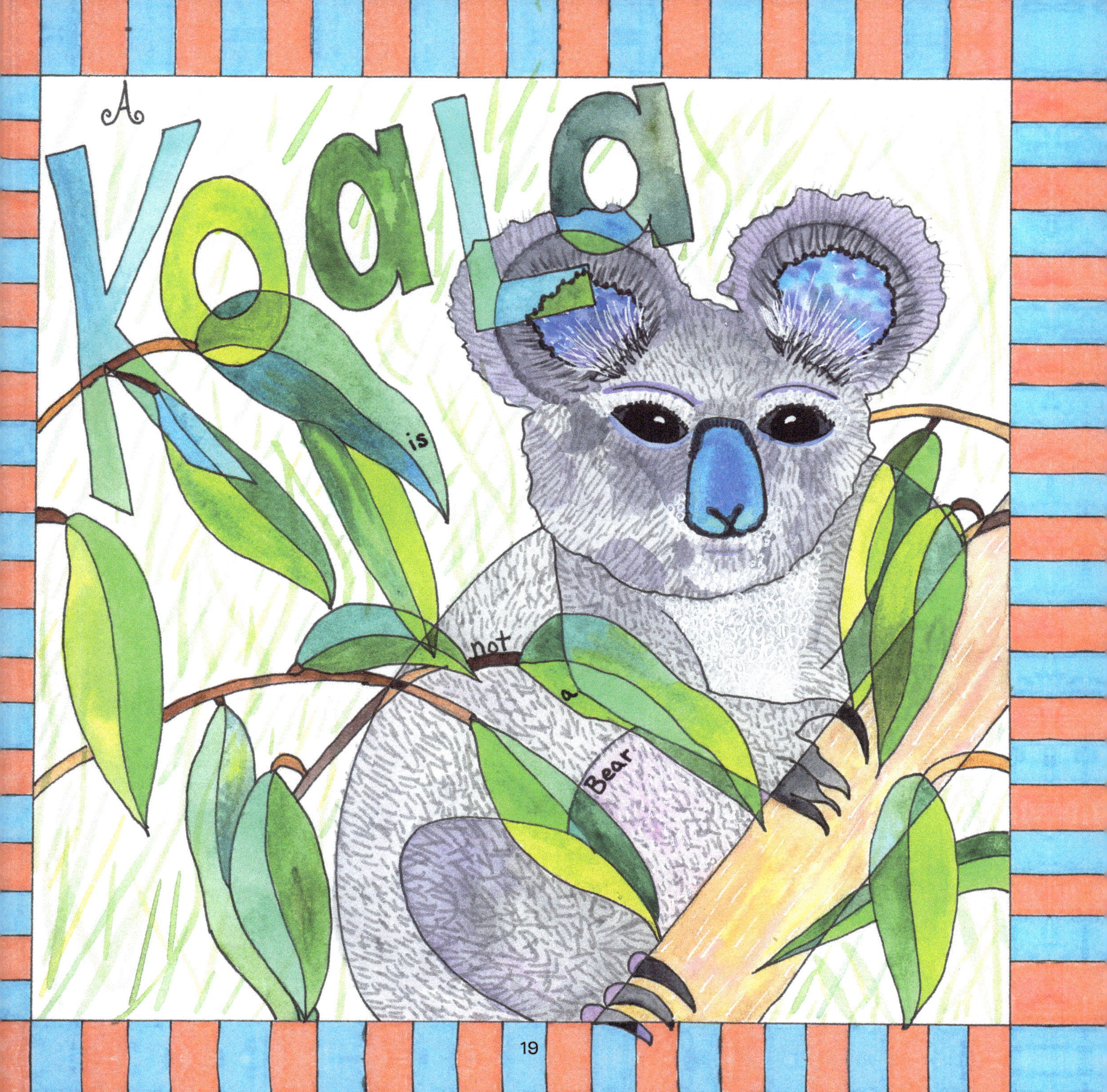

A Koala
is
not
a
Bear

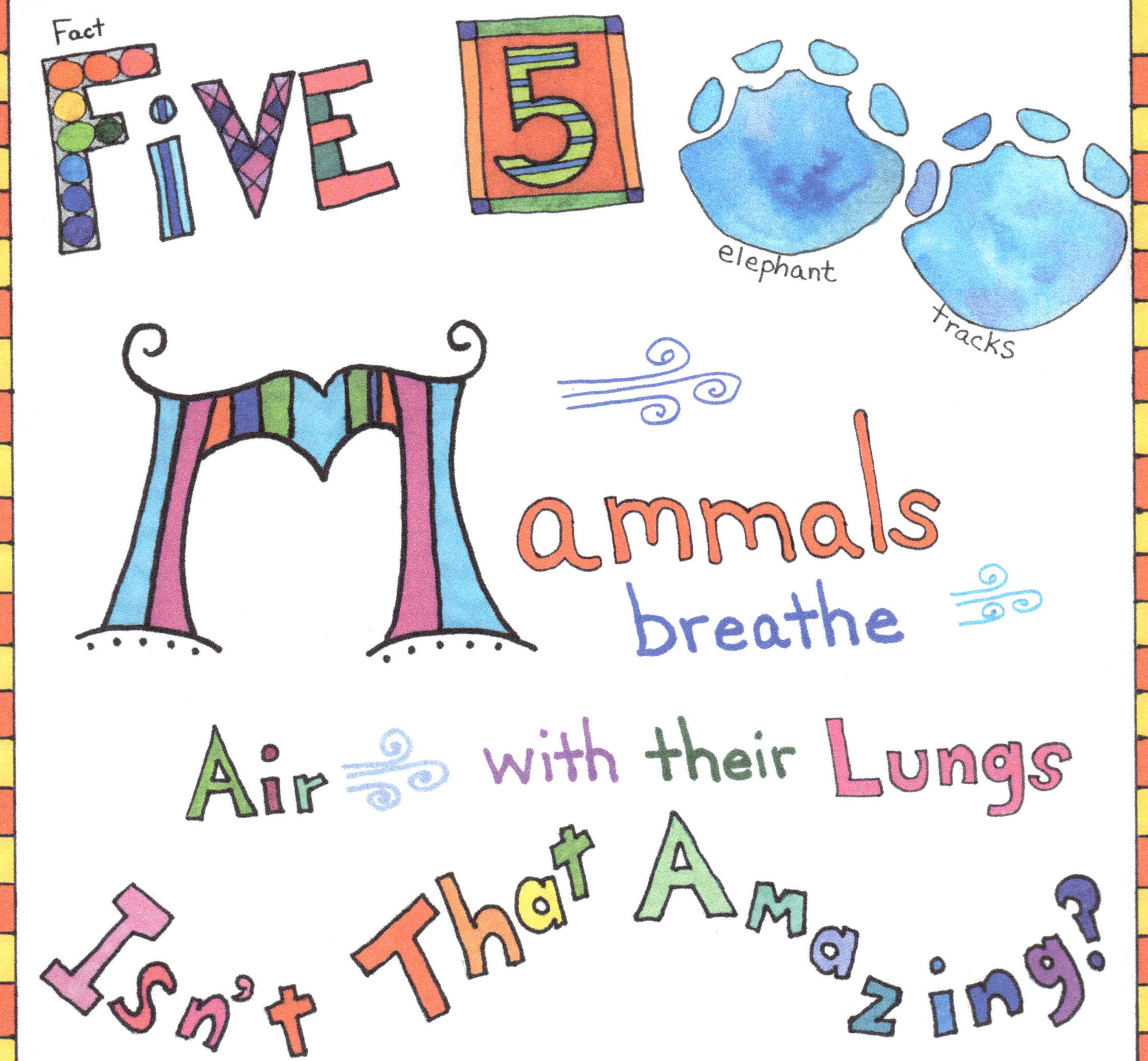

Fact
FIVE 5
elephant tracks
Mammals breathe Air with their Lungs
Isn't That Amazing?

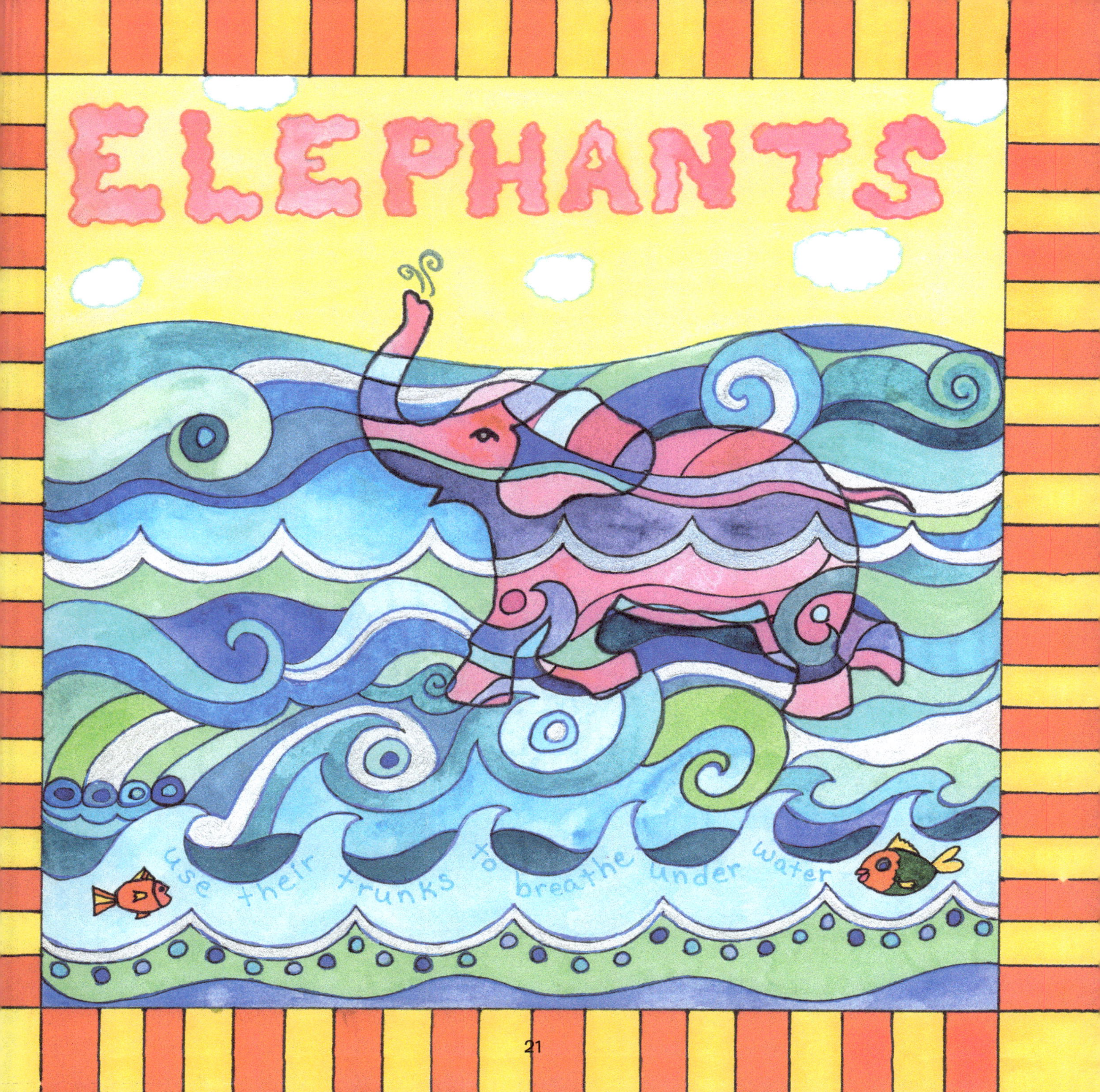

ELEPHANTS
use their trunks to breathe under water

Fact Six 6

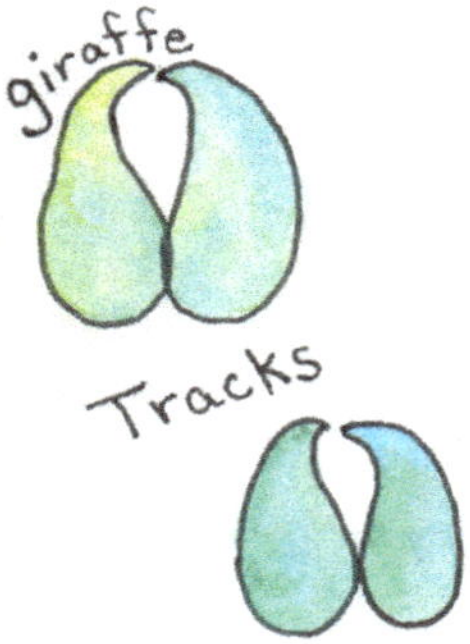
giraffe
Tracks

Mammals

have a skeleton with a back-bone.

Isn't That Amazing?

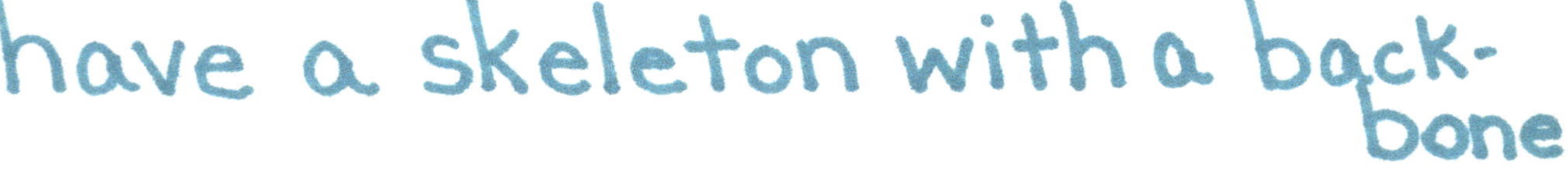

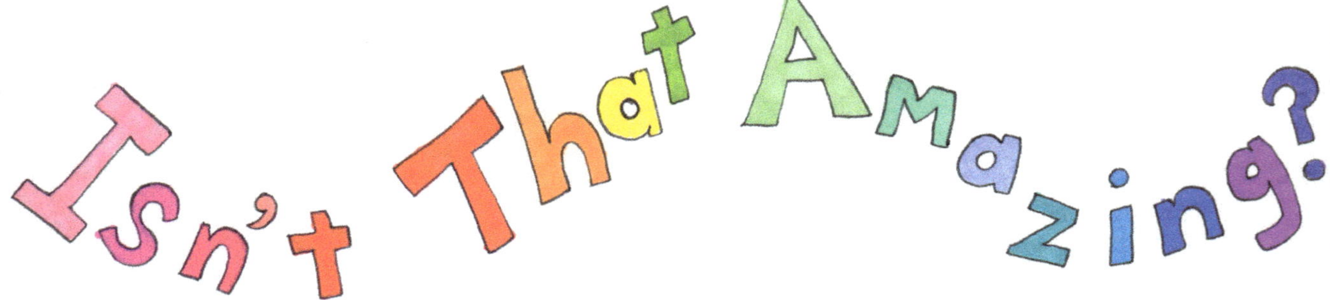

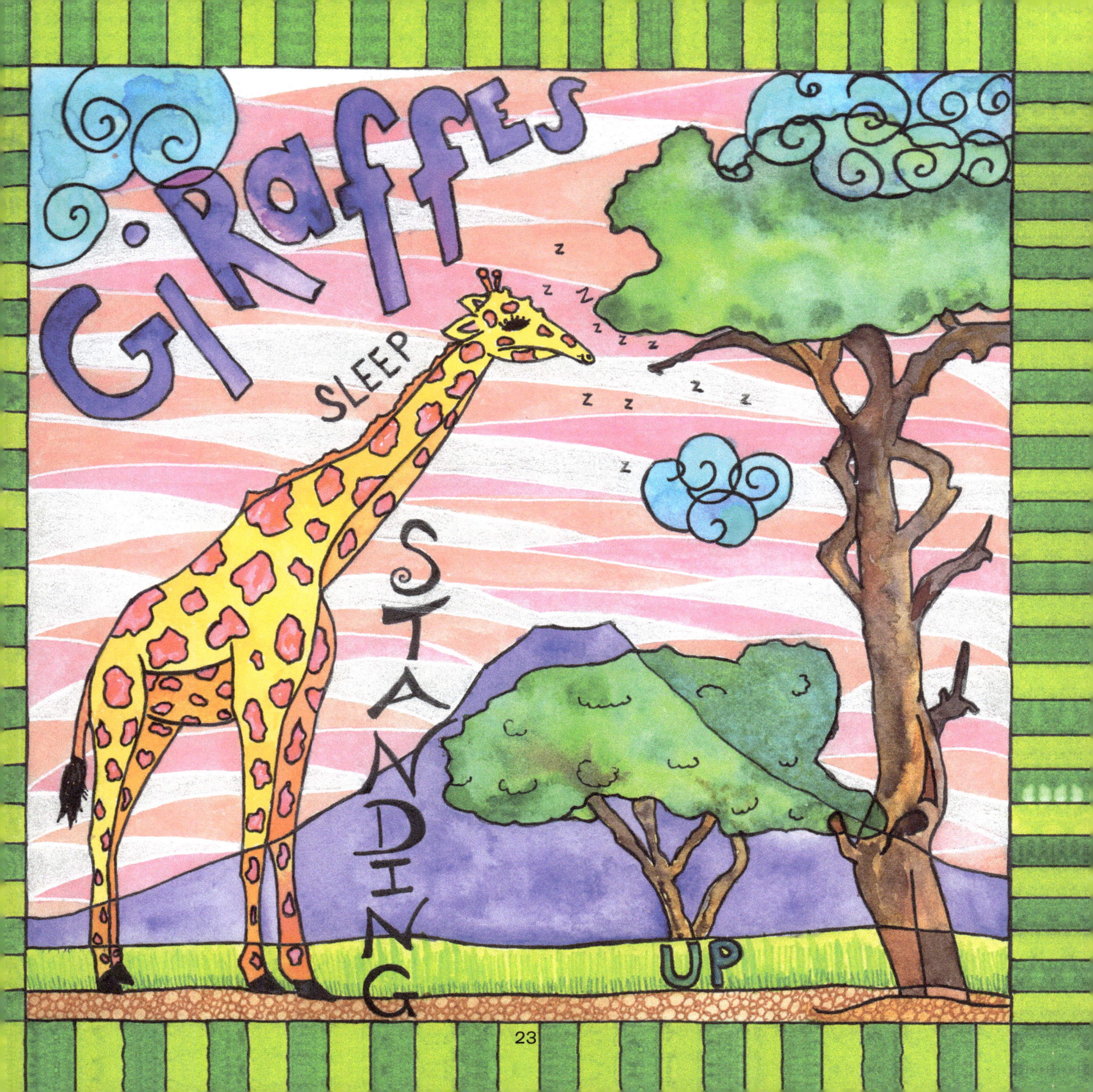

GIRAFFES
SLEEP
STANDING
UP

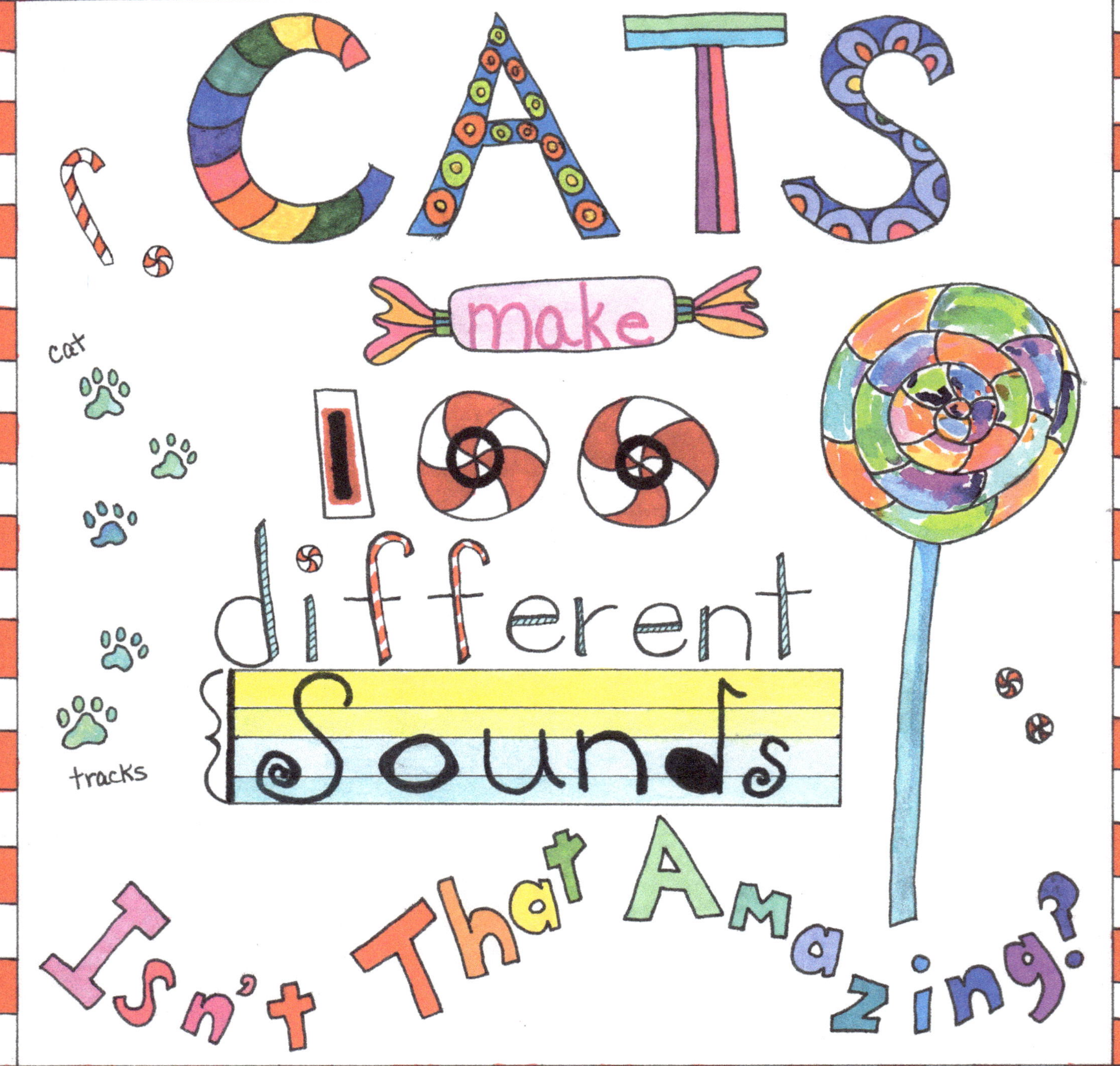

CATS
make
100
different
Sounds
Isn't That Amazing?
cat
tracks

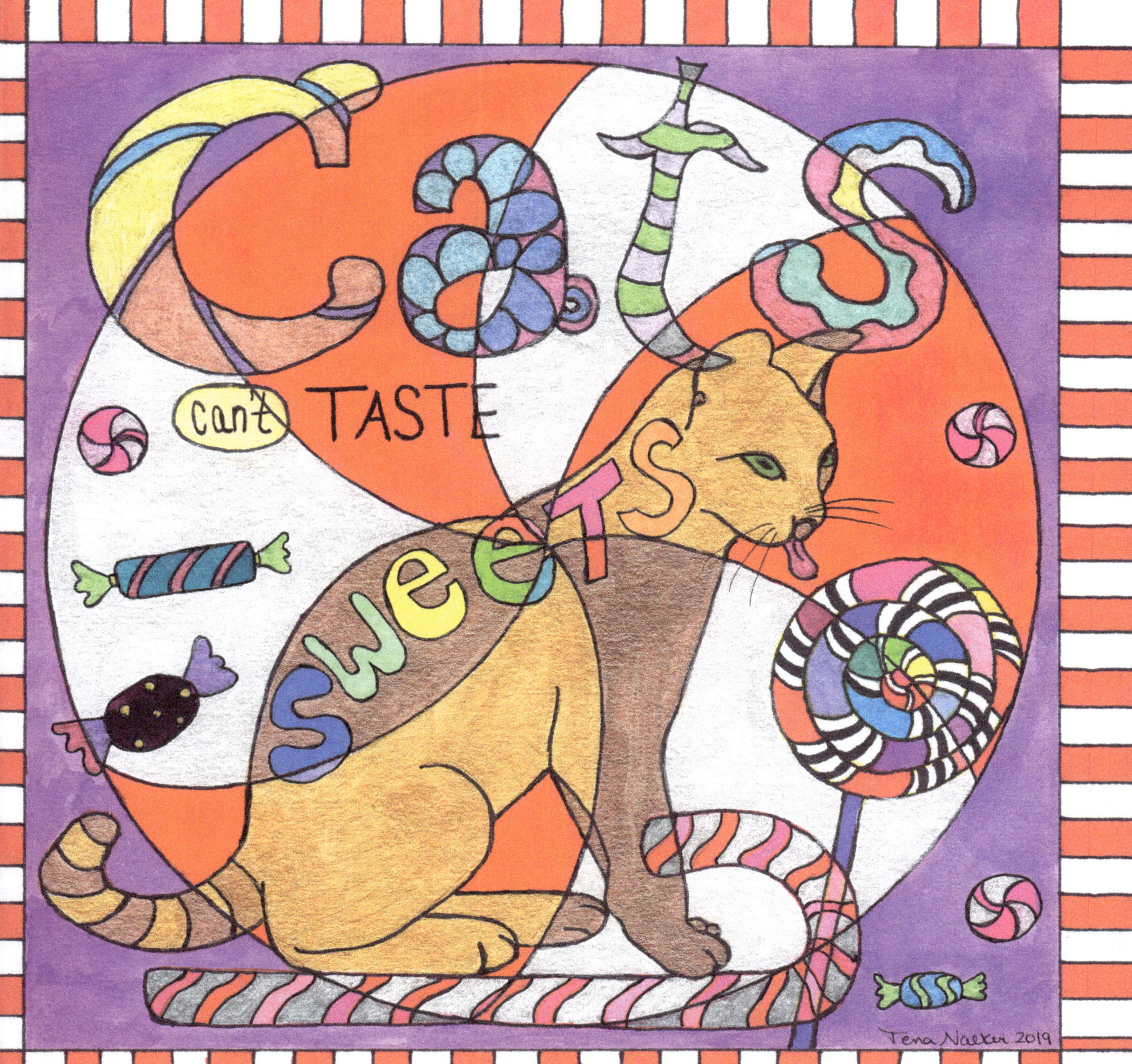

Cats
can't TASTE
sweets
Tena Naeu 2019

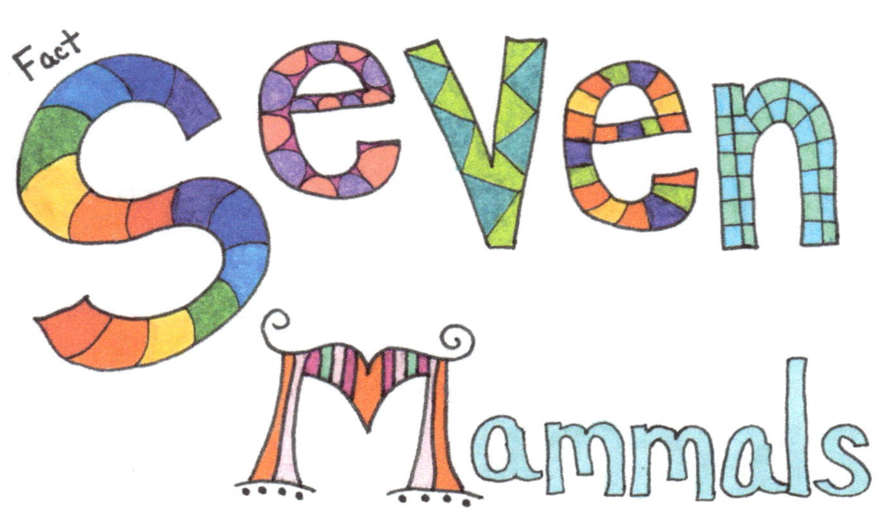
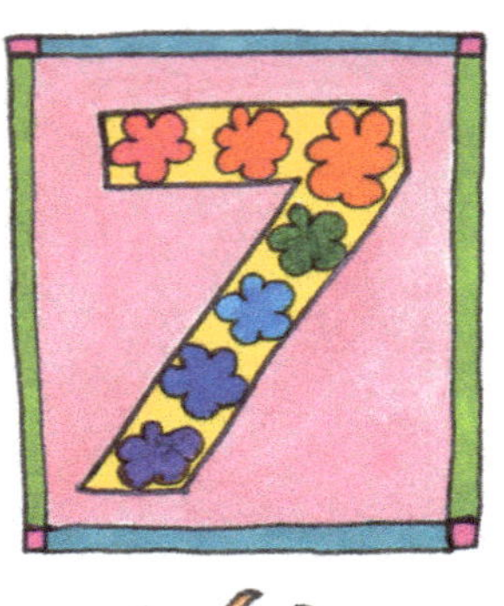
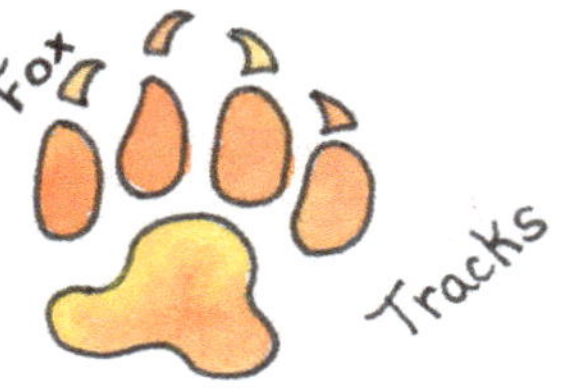

Seven 7 Mammals

can keep their body the same Temperature because they are warm-blooded.

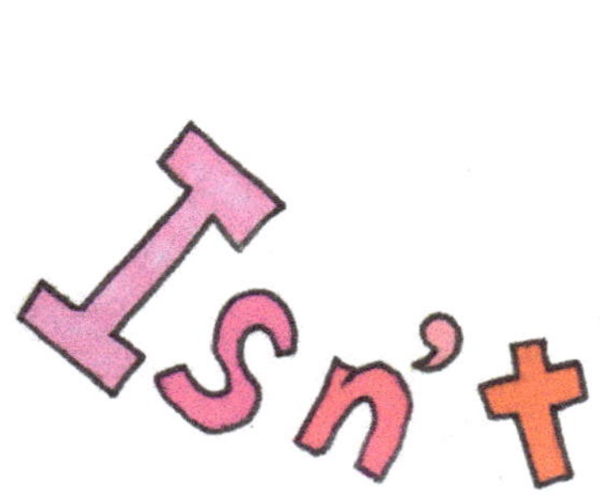
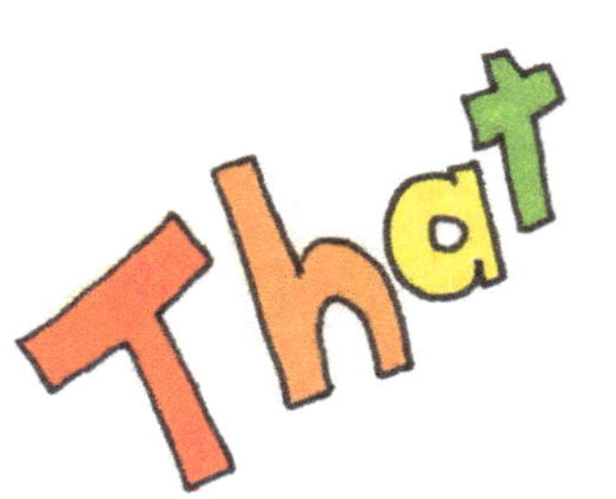
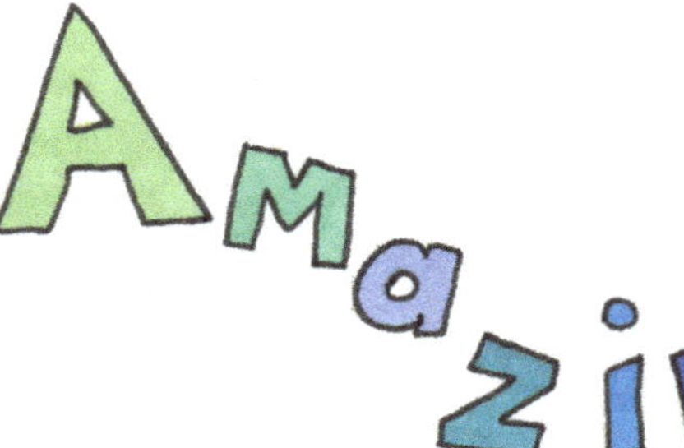

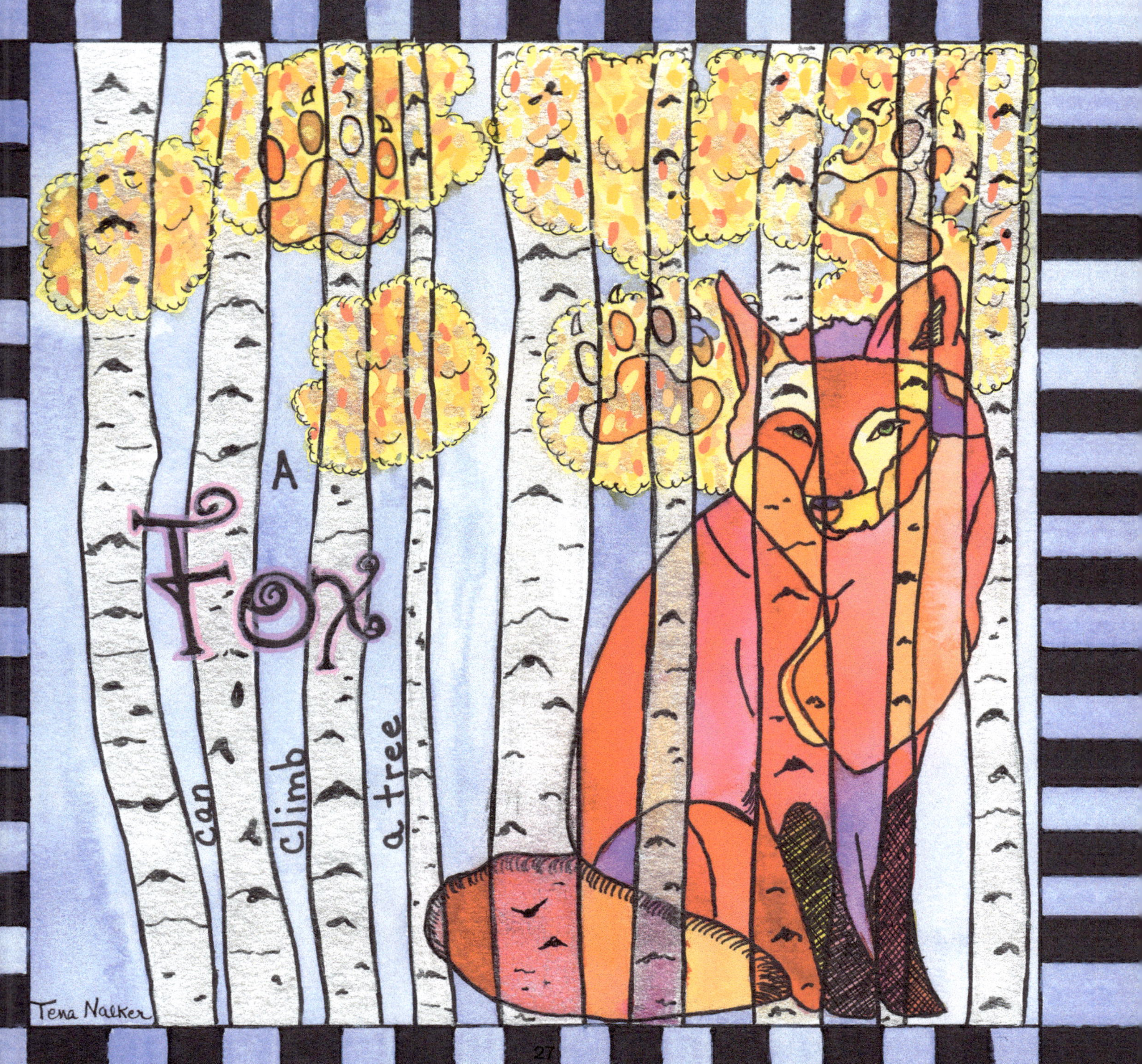
A
Fox
can
Climb
a tree
Tena Nalker

and **YOU** are

Look in a

MIRROR

a **MAMMAL** too

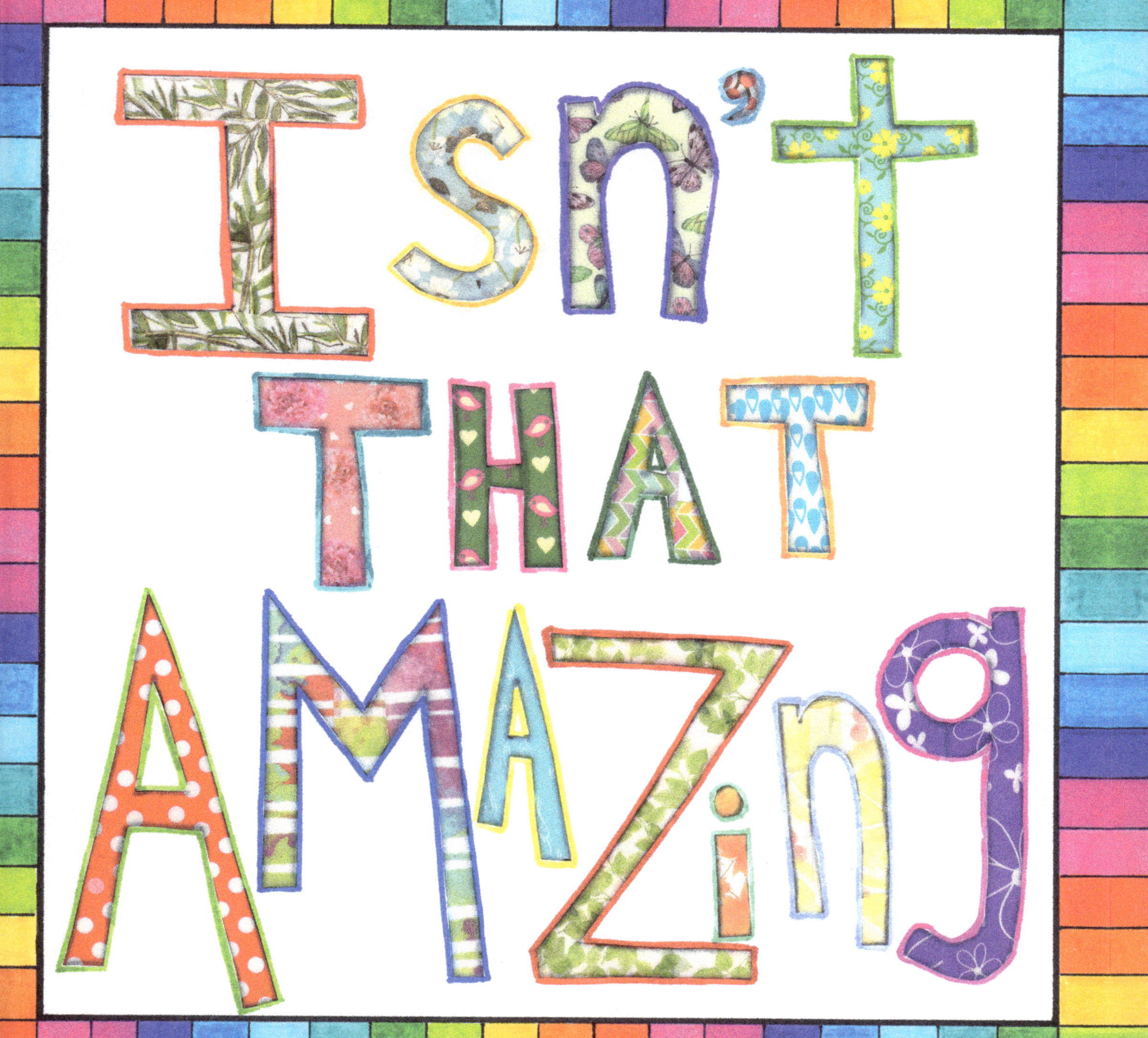

ISN'T THAT AMAZING

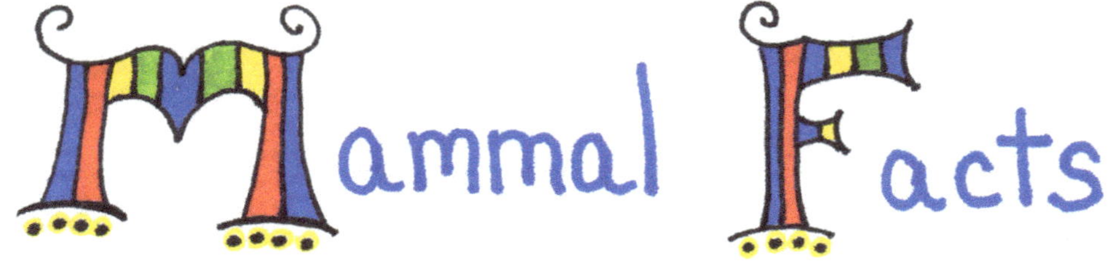

1. feed their babies milk

2. have fur or hair

3. give birth to live young

4. are very smart

5. breathe air
with their lungs

6. have a skeleton
with a backbone

7. can keep their body
the same temperature
because they are warm-blooded

Amazing Facts

- Happy cows produce more milk.
- Gorillas have fingerprints like humans.
- Gorillas eat mostly leaves and fruit.
- Jaguars are excellent climbers.
- A hedgehog has over 5000 quills on their back.
- Hedgehogs are nocturnal.
- Rabbits can have 50 babies in one year.
- Horses can smell happiness and fear.
- Horses are afraid of butterflies.
- Whales sing when they communicate.
- Koalas can only be found in eastern Australia.
- A Koala is not a bear.
- Elephants use their trunks to breathe under water.
- Giraffes sleep standing up.
- Cats make 100 different sounds.
- Cats can't taste sweets.
- A fox can climb a tree.